AF553610

# *Cumulative Student Activity Record of Clinical Experience*
# *for*
# *MSc Nursing Program*
# (Log-Book)

---

*Prepared as per the Syllabus of INC New Delhi and BFUHS Faridkot (Punjab)*

# Cumulative Student Activity Record of Clinical Experience for MSc Nursing Program (Log Book)

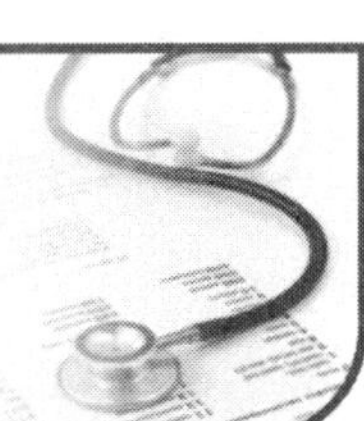

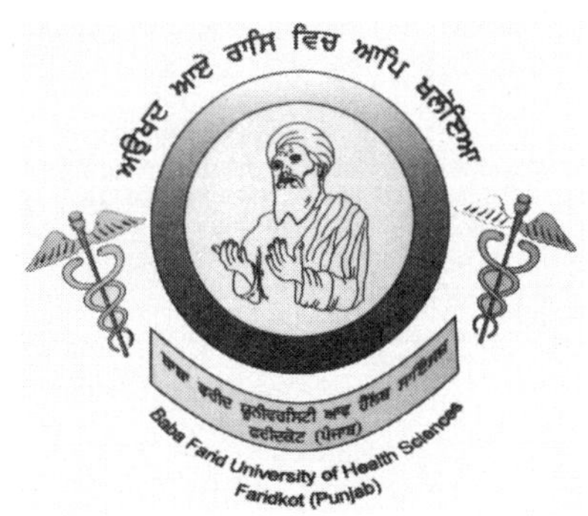


*Prof HC Rawat*
Vice Principal
University College of Nursing BFUHS Faridkot
Punjab, India

**University College of Nursing**
Baba Farid University of Health Sciences
Faridkot – 151203 Punjab, India

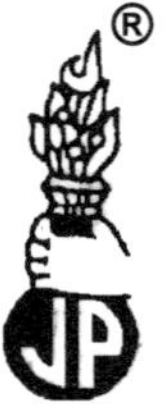

**JAYPEE BROTHERS MEDICAL PUBLISHERS (P) LTD**

**New Delhi • Panama City • London**

*Published by*
**Jaypee Brothers Medical Publishers (P) Ltd**

***Corporate Office***
4838/24 Ansari Road, Daryaganj, **New Delhi** – 110 002, India
Phone: +91-11-43574357, Fax: +91-11-43574314
Website: www.jaypeebrothers.com

***Offices in India***
- **Ahmedabad**, e-mail: ahmedabad@jaypeebrothers.com
- **Bengaluru**, e-mail: bangalore@jaypeebrothers.com
- **Chennai**, e-mail: chennai@jaypeebrothers.com
- **Delhi**, e-mail: jaypee@jaypeebrothers.com
- **Hyderabad**, e-mail: hyderabad@jaypeebrothers.com
- **Kochi**, e-mail: kochi@jaypeebrothers.com
- **Kolkata**, e-mail: kolkata@jaypeebrothers.com
- **Lucknow**, e-mail: lucknow@jaypeebrothers.com
- **Mumbai**, e-mail: mumbai@jaypeebrothers.com
- **Nagpur**, e-mail: nagpur@jaypeebrothers.com

***Overseas Offices***
- **Central America Office, Panama City, Panama,** Ph: 001-507-317-0160, e-mail: cservice@jphmedical.com, Website: www.jphmedical.com
- **Europe Office, UK,** Ph: +44 (0) 2031708910, e-mail: info@jpmedpub.com

**Cumulative Student Activity Record of Clinical Experience for MSc Nursing Program**


*First Edition:* **2012**

*ISBN:* 978-93-5025-902-3

*Typeset at:* JPBMP typesetting unit

Printed at Rajkamal Electric Press, Plot No. 2, Phase-IV, Kundli, Haryana.

# Preface

In delivering of quality nursing care to individual client and community , three major learning domains (KAP) knowledge, attitude and practice/ psychomotor skills domains are the vital/essential component for application of theories and principles in his/her area of nursing specialty , advance nursing practice and performing professional duties effectively as educator manager and researcher in the field of nursing.

The main purpose of maintaining this log book/record of Practical activities and assignment is to ensure that various activities/nursing skills has been taught by nursing faculty with expected level of satisfaction to provide nursing service to mankind, independently in their future professional career.

This practical experience Log book is a written document and very important for the post graduate students as well as for faculty member to inforce the systematic learning process and it would provide uniform learning opportunity regarding KAP by the PG students under supervision during the course.

This log book in designed according to new syllabus of MSc nursing course approved by faculty of nursing Sciences BFUHS Faridkot Punjab.

I am indeed immensely grateful thanks to prof. Raj Rani Principal University College of Nursing BFUHS Faridkot and Mr. Bhupesh Arora of Jaypee Brothers Medical Publisher's (P) Ltd. Who urged me to embark on this venture and provided all kind of assistance and encouragement to complete this clinical logbook for MSc Nursing Students.

**Prof HC Rawat**

## Students Identification Profile

Paste
Passport
Size Photograph

**Name of Student:** ______________________

**Roll No:** ______________________

**Specialty:** ______________________

**Date of Joining:** ______________________

**Father's /Husband's Name:** ______________________

**Date of Birth:** ______________________

**Permanent Address:** ______________________

______________________

______________________

______________________

**Local Guardian:**

**Address:** ______________________

______________________

______________________

**Nonsponsored/**

**Sponsored Candidate:** ______________________

**If Sponsored Affiliate with:** ______________________

______________________

______________________

# AIMS and Objectives of MSc Nursing Course

**At the end of the training program the student will be able to:**

1. Utilize/apply the concept, theories and principles drawn from nursing and allied sciences in her/his area of nursing specialty.
2. Demonstrate advance competence in practice of nursing in her/his area of nursing specialty.
3. Function effectively as educator and manage of nursing and allied health disciplines.
4. Demonstrate leadership abilities to initiate and bring about change in her/his area of practice in the health delivery system.
5. Demonstrate competence in conducting nursing research and interpret and utilize the findings of health related research.
6. Demonstrate interest in continued learning for personal and professional advancement.

# Activity Record of Clinical Experience – Ist Year

## Monthly Posting Record

**Month and year** ________________________________________

**Area of posting** ________________________________________

Work done in posting area: (Type of patient nursed, Patient care activities, Assignments, Teaching, Management, Research)

| Activities | |
|---|---|
| | |
| | |
| | |
| | |
| | |
| | |
| | |

**Skills Observed/Carried Out**

| S. No. | Skills | Observed No. of times with dates | Carried out No. of times with dates | Remarks |
|---|---|---|---|---|
| | | | | |
| | | | | |
| | | | | |
| | | | | |
| | | | | |
| | | | | |
| | | | | |
| | | | | |
| | | | | |
| | | | | |
| | | | | |
| | | | | |
| | | | | |

**Leave Availed** ________________________________________

**Remarks by Faculty** ________________________________________

**Signature of Faculty**

*One page to be used for each month of posting

## Monthly Posting Record

**Month and year** ________________________________________

**Area of posting** ________________________________________

Work done in posting area: (Type of patient nursed, Patient care activities, Assignments, Teaching, Management, Research)

| Activities | |
|---|---|
| | |
| | |
| | |
| | |
| | |
| | |
| | |

**Skills Observed/Carried Out**

| S. No. | Skills | Observed No. of times with dates | Carried out No. of times with dates | Remarks |
|---|---|---|---|---|
| | | | | |
| | | | | |
| | | | | |
| | | | | |
| | | | | |
| | | | | |
| | | | | |
| | | | | |
| | | | | |
| | | | | |
| | | | | |
| | | | | |
| | | | | |

**Leave Availed** ________________________________________

**Remarks by Faculty** ________________________________________

**Signature of Faculty**

*One page to be used for each month of posting

## Monthly Posting Record

**Month and year** ____________________

**Area of posting** ____________________

Work done in posting area: (Type of patient nursed, Patient care activities, Assignments, Teaching, Management, Research)

| Activities | |
|---|---|
| | |
| | |
| | |
| | |
| | |
| | |
| | |

**Skills Observed/Carried Out**

| S. No. | Skills | Observed No. of times with dates | Carried out No. of times with dates | Remarks |
|---|---|---|---|---|
| | | | | |
| | | | | |
| | | | | |
| | | | | |
| | | | | |
| | | | | |
| | | | | |
| | | | | |
| | | | | |
| | | | | |
| | | | | |
| | | | | |
| | | | | |

**Leave Availed** ____________________

**Remarks by Faculty** ____________________

**Signature of Faculty**

*One page to be used for each month of posting

## Monthly Posting Record

**Month and year** ___________________________

**Area of posting** ___________________________

Work done in posting area: (Type of patient nursed, Patient care activities, Assignments, Teaching, Management, Research)

| Activities | |
|---|---|
| | |
| | |
| | |
| | |
| | |
| | |
| | |

**Skills Observed/Carried Out**

| S. No. | Skills | Observed No. of times with dates | Carried out No. of times with dates | Remarks |
|---|---|---|---|---|
| | | | | |
| | | | | |
| | | | | |
| | | | | |
| | | | | |
| | | | | |
| | | | | |
| | | | | |
| | | | | |
| | | | | |
| | | | | |
| | | | | |
| | | | | |

**Leave Availed** ___________________________

**Remarks by Faculty** ___________________________

**Signature of Faculty**

*One page to be used for each month of posting

## Monthly Posting Record

**Month and year** ____________________

**Area of posting** ____________________

Work done in posting area: (Type of patient nursed, Patient care activities, Assignments, Teaching, Management, Research)

| Activities | |
|---|---|
| | |
| | |
| | |
| | |
| | |
| | |
| | |

**Skills Observed/Carried Out**

| S. No. | Skills | Observed No. of times with dates | Carried out No. of times with dates | Remarks |
|---|---|---|---|---|
| | | | | |
| | | | | |
| | | | | |
| | | | | |
| | | | | |
| | | | | |
| | | | | |
| | | | | |
| | | | | |
| | | | | |
| | | | | |
| | | | | |
| | | | | |

**Leave Availed** ____________________

**Remarks by Faculty** ____________________

**Signature of Faculty**

*One page to be used for each month of posting

## Monthly Posting Record

**Month and year** ____________________

**Area of posting** ____________________

Work done in posting area: (Type of patient nursed, Patient care activities, Assignments, Teaching, Management, Research)

| Activities | |
|---|---|
| | |
| | |
| | |
| | |
| | |
| | |
| | |

**Skills Observed/Carried Out**

| S. No. | Skills | Observed No. of times with dates | Carried out No. of times with dates | Remarks |
|---|---|---|---|---|
| | | | | |
| | | | | |
| | | | | |
| | | | | |
| | | | | |
| | | | | |
| | | | | |
| | | | | |
| | | | | |
| | | | | |
| | | | | |
| | | | | |
| | | | | |

**Leave Availed** ____________________

**Remarks by Faculty** ____________________

**Signature of Faculty**

*One page to be used for each month of posting

## Monthly Posting Record

**Month and year** ____________________

**Area of posting** ____________________

Work done in posting area: (Type of patient nursed, Patient care activities, Assignments, Teaching, Management, Research)

| Activities | |
|---|---|
| | |
| | |
| | |
| | |
| | |
| | |
| | |

**Skills Observed/Carried Out**

| S. No. | Skills | Observed No. of times with dates | Carried out No. of times with dates | Remarks |
|---|---|---|---|---|
| | | | | |
| | | | | |
| | | | | |
| | | | | |
| | | | | |
| | | | | |
| | | | | |
| | | | | |
| | | | | |
| | | | | |
| | | | | |
| | | | | |
| | | | | |

**Leave Availed** ____________________

**Remarks by Faculty** ____________________

**Signature of Faculty**

*One page to be used for each month of posting

## Monthly Posting Record

**Month and year** ______________________________

**Area of posting** ______________________________

Work done in posting area: (Type of patient nursed, Patient care activities, Assignments, Teaching, Management, Research)

| Activities | |
|---|---|
| | |
| | |
| | |
| | |
| | |
| | |
| | |

**Skills Observed/Carried Out**

| S. No. | Skills | Observed No. of times with dates | Carried out No. of times with dates | Remarks |
|---|---|---|---|---|
| | | | | |
| | | | | |
| | | | | |
| | | | | |
| | | | | |
| | | | | |
| | | | | |
| | | | | |
| | | | | |
| | | | | |
| | | | | |
| | | | | |
| | | | | |

**Leave Availed** ______________________________

**Remarks by Faculty** ______________________________

**Signature of Faculty**

*One page to be used for each month of posting

## Monthly Posting Record

**Month and year** ______________________

**Area of posting** ______________________

Work done in posting area: (Type of patient nursed, Patient care activities, Assignments, Teaching, Management, Research)

| Activities | |
|---|---|
| | |
| | |
| | |
| | |
| | |
| | |
| | |

**Skills Observed/Carried Out**

| S. No. | Skills | Observed No. of times with dates | Carried out No. of times with dates | Remarks |
|---|---|---|---|---|
| | | | | |
| | | | | |
| | | | | |
| | | | | |
| | | | | |
| | | | | |
| | | | | |
| | | | | |
| | | | | |
| | | | | |
| | | | | |
| | | | | |
| | | | | |

**Leave Availed** ______________________

**Remarks by Faculty** ______________________

**Signature of Faculty**

*One page to be used for each month of posting

# Monthly Posting Record

**Month and year** ______________________________

**Area of posting** ______________________________

Work done in posting area: (Type of patient nursed, Patient care activities, Assignments, Teaching, Management, Research)

| Activities | |
|---|---|
| | |
| | |
| | |
| | |
| | |
| | |
| | |

**Skills Observed/Carried Out**

| S. No. | Skills | Observed No. of times with dates | Carried out No. of times with dates | Remarks |
|---|---|---|---|---|
| | | | | |
| | | | | |
| | | | | |
| | | | | |
| | | | | |
| | | | | |
| | | | | |
| | | | | |
| | | | | |
| | | | | |
| | | | | |
| | | | | |
| | | | | |

**Leave Availed** ______________________________

**Remarks by Faculty** ______________________________

**Signature of Faculty**

*One page to be used for each month of posting

## Monthly Posting Record

**Month and year** ____________________

**Area of posting** ____________________

Work done in posting area: (Type of patient nursed, Patient care activities, Assignments, Teaching, Management, Research)

| Activities | |
|---|---|
| | |
| | |
| | |
| | |
| | |
| | |
| | |

**Skills Observed/Carried Out**

| S. No. | Skills | Observed No. of times with dates | Carried out No. of times with dates | Remarks |
|---|---|---|---|---|
| | | | | |
| | | | | |
| | | | | |
| | | | | |
| | | | | |
| | | | | |
| | | | | |
| | | | | |
| | | | | |
| | | | | |
| | | | | |
| | | | | |
| | | | | |

**Leave Availed** ____________________

**Remarks by Faculty** ____________________

**Signature of Faculty**

*One page to be used for each month of posting

## Monthly Posting Record

**Month and year** ____________________

**Area of posting** ____________________

Work done in posting area: (Type of patient nursed, Patient care activities, Assignments, Teaching, Management, Research)

| Activities | |
|---|---|
| | |
| | |
| | |
| | |
| | |
| | |
| | |

**Skills Observed/Carried Out**

| S. No. | Skills | Observed No. of times with dates | Carried out No. of times with dates | Remarks |
|---|---|---|---|---|
| | | | | |
| | | | | |
| | | | | |
| | | | | |
| | | | | |
| | | | | |
| | | | | |
| | | | | |
| | | | | |
| | | | | |
| | | | | |
| | | | | |
| | | | | |

**Leave Availed** ____________________

**Remarks by Faculty** ____________________

**Signature of Faculty**

*One page to be used for each month of posting

## Monthly Posting Record

**Month and year** ________________________________________

**Area of posting** ________________________________________

Work done in posting area: (Type of patient nursed, Patient care activities, Assignments, Teaching, Management, Research)

| Activities | |
|---|---|
| | |
| | |
| | |
| | |
| | |
| | |
| | |

**Skills Observed/Carried Out**

| S. No. | Skills | Observed No. of times with dates | Carried out No. of times with dates | Remarks |
|---|---|---|---|---|
| | | | | |
| | | | | |
| | | | | |
| | | | | |
| | | | | |
| | | | | |
| | | | | |
| | | | | |
| | | | | |
| | | | | |
| | | | | |
| | | | | |
| | | | | |

**Leave Availed** ________________________________________

**Remarks by Faculty** ________________________________________

**Signature of Faculty**

*One page to be used for each month of posting

## Monthly Posting Record

**Month and year** ______________________________

**Area of posting** ______________________________

Work done in posting area: (Type of patient nursed, Patient care activities, Assignments, Teaching, Management, Research)

| Activities | |
|---|---|
| | |
| | |
| | |
| | |
| | |
| | |
| | |

**Skills Observed/Carried Out**

| S. No. | Skills | Observed No. of times with dates | Carried out No. of times with dates | Remarks |
|---|---|---|---|---|
| | | | | |
| | | | | |
| | | | | |
| | | | | |
| | | | | |
| | | | | |
| | | | | |
| | | | | |
| | | | | |
| | | | | |
| | | | | |
| | | | | |
| | | | | |

**Leave Availed** ______________________________

**Remarks by Faculty** ______________________________

**Signature of Faculty**

*One page to be used for each month of posting

# Activity Record of Clinical Experience – IInd Year

## Monthly Posting Record

**Month and year** ____________________

**Area of posting** ____________________

Work done in posting area: (Type of patient nursed, Patient care activities, Assignments, Teaching, Management, Research)

| Activities | |
|---|---|
| | |
| | |
| | |
| | |
| | |
| | |
| | |

**Skills Observed/Carried Out**

| S. No. | Skills | Observed No. of times with dates | Carried out No. of times with dates | Remarks |
|---|---|---|---|---|
| | | | | |
| | | | | |
| | | | | |
| | | | | |
| | | | | |
| | | | | |
| | | | | |
| | | | | |
| | | | | |
| | | | | |
| | | | | |
| | | | | |
| | | | | |

**Leave Availed** ____________________

**Remarks by Faculty** ____________________

**Signature of Faculty**

*One page to be used for each month of posting

## Monthly Posting Record

**Month and year** ____________________

**Area of posting** ____________________

Work done in posting area: (Type of patient nursed, Patient care activities, Assignments, Teaching, Management, Research)

| Activities | |
|---|---|
| | |
| | |
| | |
| | |
| | |
| | |
| | |

**Skills Observed/Carried Out**

| S. No. | Skills | Observed No. of times with dates | Carried out No. of times with dates | Remarks |
|---|---|---|---|---|
| | | | | |
| | | | | |
| | | | | |
| | | | | |
| | | | | |
| | | | | |
| | | | | |
| | | | | |
| | | | | |
| | | | | |
| | | | | |
| | | | | |
| | | | | |

**Leave Availed** ____________________

**Remarks by Faculty** ____________________

**Signature of Faculty**

*One page to be used for each month of posting

## Monthly Posting Record

**Month and year** ______________________________

**Area of posting** ______________________________

Work done in posting area: (Type of patient nursed, Patient care activities, Assignments, Teaching, Management, Research)

| Activities | |
|---|---|
| | |
| | |
| | |
| | |
| | |
| | |
| | |

**Skills Observed/Carried Out**

| S. No. | Skills | Observed No. of times with dates | Carried out No. of times with dates | Remarks |
|---|---|---|---|---|
| | | | | |
| | | | | |
| | | | | |
| | | | | |
| | | | | |
| | | | | |
| | | | | |
| | | | | |
| | | | | |
| | | | | |
| | | | | |
| | | | | |
| | | | | |

**Leave Availed** ______________________________

**Remarks by Faculty** ______________________________

**Signature of Faculty**

*One page to be used for each month of posting

## Monthly Posting Record

**Month and year** ______________________________

**Area of posting** ______________________________

Work done in posting area: (Type of patient nursed, Patient care activities, Assignments, Teaching, Management, Research)

| Activities | |
|---|---|
| | |
| | |
| | |
| | |
| | |
| | |
| | |

**Skills Observed/Carried Out**

| S. No. | Skills | Observed No. of times with dates | Carried out No. of times with dates | Remarks |
|---|---|---|---|---|
| | | | | |
| | | | | |
| | | | | |
| | | | | |
| | | | | |
| | | | | |
| | | | | |
| | | | | |
| | | | | |
| | | | | |
| | | | | |
| | | | | |
| | | | | |

**Leave Availed** ______________________________

**Remarks by Faculty** ______________________________

**Signature of Faculty**

*One page to be used for each month of posting

## Monthly Posting Record

**Month and year** ____________________

**Area of posting** ____________________

Work done in posting area: (Type of patient nursed, Patient care activities, Assignments, Teaching, Management, Research)

| Activities | |
|---|---|
| | |
| | |
| | |
| | |
| | |
| | |
| | |

**Skills Observed/Carried Out**

| S. No. | Skills | Observed No. of times with dates | Carried out No. of times with dates | Remarks |
|---|---|---|---|---|
| | | | | |
| | | | | |
| | | | | |
| | | | | |
| | | | | |
| | | | | |
| | | | | |
| | | | | |
| | | | | |
| | | | | |
| | | | | |
| | | | | |
| | | | | |

**Leave Availed** ____________________

**Remarks by Faculty** ____________________

**Signature of Faculty**

*One page to be used for each month of posting

## Monthly Posting Record

**Month and year** ______________________

**Area of posting** ______________________

Work done in posting area: (Type of patient nursed, Patient care activities, Assignments, Teaching, Management, Research)

| Activities | |
|---|---|
| | |
| | |
| | |
| | |
| | |
| | |
| | |

**Skills Observed/Carried Out**

| S. No. | Skills | Observed No. of times with dates | Carried out No. of times with dates | Remarks |
|---|---|---|---|---|
| | | | | |
| | | | | |
| | | | | |
| | | | | |
| | | | | |
| | | | | |
| | | | | |
| | | | | |
| | | | | |
| | | | | |
| | | | | |
| | | | | |
| | | | | |

**Leave Availed** ______________________

**Remarks by Faculty** ______________________

**Signature of Faculty**

*One page to be used for each month of posting

## Monthly Posting Record

**Month and year** ________________________________________________

**Area of posting** ________________________________________________

Work done in posting area: (Type of patient nursed, Patient care activities, Assignments, Teaching, Management, Research)

| **Activities** | |
|---|---|
| | |
| | |
| | |
| | |
| | |
| | |
| | |

**Skills Observed/Carried Out**

| **S. No.** | **Skills** | **Observed No. of times with dates** | **Carried out No. of times with dates** | **Remarks** |
|---|---|---|---|---|
| | | | | |
| | | | | |
| | | | | |
| | | | | |
| | | | | |
| | | | | |
| | | | | |
| | | | | |
| | | | | |
| | | | | |
| | | | | |
| | | | | |
| | | | | |

**Leave Availed** ________________________________________________

**Remarks by Faculty** ________________________________________________

**Signature of Faculty**

*One page to be used for each month of posting

# Monthly Posting Record

**Month and year** ______________________________

**Area of posting** ______________________________

Work done in posting area: (Type of patient nursed, Patient care activities, Assignments, Teaching, Management, Research)

| Activities | |
|---|---|
| | |
| | |
| | |
| | |
| | |
| | |
| | |

**Skills Observed/Carried Out**

| S. No. | Skills | Observed No. of times with dates | Carried out No. of times with dates | Remarks |
|---|---|---|---|---|
| | | | | |
| | | | | |
| | | | | |
| | | | | |
| | | | | |
| | | | | |
| | | | | |
| | | | | |
| | | | | |
| | | | | |
| | | | | |
| | | | | |
| | | | | |

**Leave Availed** ______________________________

**Remarks by Faculty** ______________________________

**Signature of Faculty**

*One page to be used for each month of posting

## Monthly Posting Record

**Month and year** ____________________

**Area of posting** ____________________

Work done in posting area: (Type of patient nursed, Patient care activities, Assignments, Teaching, Management, Research)

| Activities | |
|---|---|
| | |
| | |
| | |
| | |
| | |
| | |
| | |

**Skills Observed/Carried Out**

| S. No. | Skills | Observed No. of times with dates | Carried out No. of times with dates | Remarks |
|---|---|---|---|---|
| | | | | |
| | | | | |
| | | | | |
| | | | | |
| | | | | |
| | | | | |
| | | | | |
| | | | | |
| | | | | |
| | | | | |
| | | | | |
| | | | | |
| | | | | |

**Leave Availed** ____________________

**Remarks by Faculty** ____________________

**Signature of Faculty**

*One page to be used for each month of posting

## Monthly Posting Record

**Month and year** ____________________

**Area of posting** ____________________

Work done in posting area: (Type of patient nursed, Patient care activities, Assignments, Teaching, Management, Research)

| Activities | |
|---|---|
| | |
| | |
| | |
| | |
| | |
| | |
| | |

**Skills Observed/Carried Out**

| S. No. | Skills | Observed No. of times with dates | Carried out No. of times with dates | Remarks |
|---|---|---|---|---|
| | | | | |
| | | | | |
| | | | | |
| | | | | |
| | | | | |
| | | | | |
| | | | | |
| | | | | |
| | | | | |
| | | | | |
| | | | | |
| | | | | |
| | | | | |

**Leave Availed** ____________________

**Remarks by Faculty** ____________________

**Signature of Faculty**

*One page to be used for each month of posting

# Monthly Posting Record

**Month and year** ______________________________

**Area of posting** ______________________________

Work done in posting area: (Type of patient nursed, Patient care activities, Assignments, Teaching, Management, Research)

| Activities | |
|---|---|
| | |
| | |
| | |
| | |
| | |
| | |
| | |

**Skills Observed/Carried Out**

| S. No. | Skills | Observed No. of times with dates | Carried out No. of times with dates | Remarks |
|---|---|---|---|---|
| | | | | |
| | | | | |
| | | | | |
| | | | | |
| | | | | |
| | | | | |
| | | | | |
| | | | | |
| | | | | |
| | | | | |
| | | | | |
| | | | | |
| | | | | |

**Leave Availed** ______________________________

**Remarks by Faculty** ______________________________

**Signature of Faculty**

*One page to be used for each month of posting

## Monthly Posting Record

**Month and year** ______________________________

**Area of posting** ______________________________

Work done in posting area: (Type of patient nursed, Patient care activities, Assignments, Teaching, Management, Research)

| Activities | |
|---|---|
| | |
| | |
| | |
| | |
| | |
| | |
| | |

**Skills Observed/Carried Out**

| S. No. | Skills | Observed No. of times with dates | Carried out No. of times with dates | Remarks |
|---|---|---|---|---|
| | | | | |
| | | | | |
| | | | | |
| | | | | |
| | | | | |
| | | | | |
| | | | | |
| | | | | |
| | | | | |
| | | | | |
| | | | | |
| | | | | |
| | | | | |

**Leave Availed** ______________________________

**Remarks by Faculty** ______________________________

**Signature of Faculty**

*One page to be used for each month of posting

## Monthly Posting Record

**Month and year** ______________________________

**Area of posting** ______________________________

Work done in posting area: (Type of patient nursed, Patient care activities, Assignments, Teaching, Management, Research)

| Activities | |
|---|---|
| | |
| | |
| | |
| | |
| | |
| | |
| | |

**Skills Observed/Carried Out**

| S. No. | Skills | Observed No. of times with dates | Carried out No. of times with dates | Remarks |
|---|---|---|---|---|
| | | | | |
| | | | | |
| | | | | |
| | | | | |
| | | | | |
| | | | | |
| | | | | |
| | | | | |
| | | | | |
| | | | | |
| | | | | |
| | | | | |
| | | | | |

**Leave Availed** ______________________________

**Remarks by Faculty** ______________________________

**Signature of Faculty**

*One page to be used for each month of posting

## Monthly Posting Record

**Month and year** ____________________

**Area of posting** ____________________

Work done in posting area: (Type of patient nursed, Patient care activities, Assignments, Teaching, Management, Research)

| Activities | |
|---|---|
| | |
| | |
| | |
| | |
| | |
| | |
| | |

**Skills Observed/Carried Out**

| S. No. | Skills | Observed No. of times with dates | Carried out No. of times with dates | Remarks |
|---|---|---|---|---|
| | | | | |
| | | | | |
| | | | | |
| | | | | |
| | | | | |
| | | | | |
| | | | | |
| | | | | |
| | | | | |
| | | | | |
| | | | | |
| | | | | |
| | | | | |

**Leave Availed** ____________________

**Remarks by Faculty** ____________________

**Signature of Faculty**

*One page to be used for each month of posting

## Seminars – Advanced Nursing Practices

| Date | Topic | Presented | Attended |
|---|---|---|---|
| | | | |

## Seminars – Advanced Nursing Practices

| Date | Topic | Presented | Attended |
|---|---|---|---|
| | | | |

# Seminars – Advanced Nursing Practices

| Date | Topic | Presented | Attended |
|---|---|---|---|
| | | | |

## Seminars – Advanced Nursing Practices

| Date | Topic | Presented | Attended |
|---|---|---|---|
| | | | |

## Seminars – Advanced Nursing Practices

| Date | Topic | Presented | Attended |
|---|---|---|---|
| | | | |

## Seminars – Advanced Nursing Practices

| Date | Topic | Presented | Attended |
|---|---|---|---|
| | | | |

## Seminars – Nursing Educations

| Date | Topic | Presented | Attended |
| --- | --- | --- | --- |
| | | | |

## Seminars – Nursing Educations

| Date | Topic | Presented | Attended |
|---|---|---|---|
| | | | |

## Seminars – Clinical Speciality I

| Date | Topic | Presented | Attended |
|---|---|---|---|
| | | | |

# Seminars – Clinical Speciality I

| Date | Topic | Presented | Attended |
|---|---|---|---|
| | | | |

## UG Lectures

(Classroom and Clinical Teaching)

| Topic | Date and Time | Taken by | Lectures | | Initials by concerned faculty |
|---|---|---|---|---|---|
| | | | No. Held | No. Attended | |
| | | | | | |

## UG Lectures

(Classroom and Clinical Teaching)

| Topic | Date and Time | Taken by | Lectures | | Initials by concerned faculty |
|---|---|---|---|---|---|
| | | | No. Held | No. Attended | |
| | | | | | |

# UG Lectures

(Classroom and Clinical Teaching)

| Topic | Date and Time | Taken by | Lectures | | Initials by concerned faculty |
|---|---|---|---|---|---|
| | | | No. Held | No. Attended | |
| | | | | | |

## UG Lectures

(Classroom and Clinical Teaching)

| Topic | Date and Time | Taken by | Lectures | | Initials by concerned faculty |
|---|---|---|---|---|---|
| | | | No. Held | No. Attended | |
| | | | | | |

# Journal Club

| Date | Area/Topic & Journal | Presented | Attended |
|---|---|---|---|
| | | | |

## Journal Club

| Date | Area/Topic & Journal | Presented | Attended |
|---|---|---|---|
| | | | |

# Journal Club

| Date | Area/Topic & Journal | Presented | Attended |
|---|---|---|---|
| | | | |

## Journal Club

| Date | Area/Topic & Journal | Presented | Attended |
|---|---|---|---|
| | | | |

# Journal Club

| Date | Area/Topic & Journal | Presented | Attended |
|---|---|---|---|
| | | | |

## Journal Club

| Date | Area/Topic & Journal | Presented | Attended |
|---|---|---|---|
| | | | |

## In Service Education/Workshop Organized

**Title** ______________________________

______________________________

**Group** ______________________ **Number** ______________

**Duration** ______________________________

**Areas of Contribution** ______________________________

______________________________

______________________________

______________________________

______________________________

______________________________

**Remarks** **Signature of Faculty**

## In Service Education/Workshop Organized

**Title** ____________________

____________________

**Group** ____________________ **Number** ____________________

**Duration** ____________________

**Areas of Contribution** ____________________

____________________

____________________

____________________

____________________

____________________

**Remarks**

**Signature of Faculty**

# Practical Examination MSc Nursing Ist year

## Clinical – Specialty – I

**Signature of Internal Examiner**
**Date:**

**Signature of External Examiner**
**Date:**

**Signature of Internal Examiner**
**Date:**

**Signature of External Examiner**
**Date:**

## Nursing Education

**Signature of Internal Examiner**
**Date:**

**Signature of External Examiner**
**Date:**

**Signature of Internal Examiner**
**Date:**

**Signature of External Examiner**
**Date:**

## Seminars – Clinical Speciality II

| Date | Topic | Presented | Attended |
|---|---|---|---|
| | | | |

## Seminars – Clinical Speciality II

| Date | Topic | Presented | Attended |
|---|---|---|---|
| | | | |

## Seminars – Nursing Management

| Date | Topic | Presented | Attended |
| --- | --- | --- | --- |
| | | | |

# Seminars – Nursing Management

| Date | Topic | Presented | Attended |
|---|---|---|---|
| | | | |

# Scientific Contributions

**CNE/Workshop Attended/Organized**

| S. No. | Name of CNE/Workshop | Held at | Date |
|---|---|---|---|
| | | | |
| | | | |
| | | | |
| | | | |
| | | | |

**Conferences Attended**

| S. No. | Name of CNE/Workshop/Conference | Held at | Date |
|---|---|---|---|
| | | | |
| | | | |
| | | | |
| | | | |
| | | | |

**Publications:** ____________________

____________________

**Awards:** ____________________

____________________

## In Service Education/Workshop Organized

**Title** ____________________

____________________

**Group** ____________________ **Number** ____________________

**Duration** ____________________

**Areas of Contribution** ____________________

____________________

____________________

____________________

____________________

____________________

**Remarks**

**Signature of Faculty**

# Thesis/Dissertation

**Topic:** ______________________________

______________________________

______________________________

**Guide:** ______________________________

**Co Guides:**

1. ______________________________
2. ______________________________
3. ______________________________

**Protocol Presented on:** ______________________________

**Thesis Postings:**

1. ______________ 2. ______________

3. ______________ 4. ______________

**Progress of Thesis:**

| Years | Work Done | Signature of Guide |
|---|---|---|
| 1st | | |
| 2nd | | |

**Thesis Presentation on:** ______________________________

**Thesis Submitted on:** ______________________________

**Grading by External Examiner:** ______________________________

# Practical Examination
# MSc Nursing IInd year

## Clinical – Speciality – II

**Signature of Internal Examiner**
**Date:**

**Signature of External Examiner**
**Date:**

**Signature of Internal Examiner**
**Date:**

**Signature of External Examiner**
**Date:**

## Dissertation/Theses/Viva Voce

**Signature of Internal Examiner**
**Date:**

**Signature of External Examiner**
**Date:**

**Signature of Internal Examiner**
**Date:**

**Signature of External Examiner**
**Date:**

## Curriculum Pattern and Examination Scheme

### First Year

| Subject | Study Hours | | Theory Marks | | | Practical Marks | | | Grand Total | Duration of Paper |
|---|---|---|---|---|---|---|---|---|---|---|
| | Theory | Practical | Univ. Exam | Int. Ass. | Total | Practical | Int. Ass | Total | | |
| Advanced Nursing Practice | 150 | 200 | 75 | 25 | 100 | – | – | – | 100 | 3Hrs. |
| Nursing education | 150 | 150 | 75 | 25 | 100 | 50 | 50 | 100 | 200 | 3Hrs |
| Nursing Research & Statistics | 150 | 100 | 75 | 25 | 100 | – | – | – | 100 | 3Hrs |
| Clinical Speciality I | 150 | 650 | 75 | 25 | 100 | 100 | 100 | 200 | 300 | 3Hrs |
| **Total** | **600** | **1100** | **300** | **100** | **400** | **150** | **150** | **300** | **700** | |

## Second Year

| Subject | Study Hours | | Theory Marks | | | Practical Marks | | | Grand Total | Durat -ion of Paper |
|---|---|---|---|---|---|---|---|---|---|---|
| | Theory | Practical | Univ. Exam | Int. Ass. | Total | Practical | Int. Ass | Total | | |
| Nursing Management | 150 | 150 | 75 | 25 | 100 | _ | _ | _ | 100 | 3Hrs. |
| Nursing Research (Dissertation) | | 300 | _ | _ | _ | 100 | 100 | 200 | 200 | |
| Clinical Speciality II | 150 | 950 | 75 | 25 | 100 | 100 | 100 | 200 | 300 | 3Hrs |
| **Total** | **300** | **1400** | **150** | **100** | **200** | **200** | **200** | **400** | **600** | |

**General Remarks:** ______________________________

______________________________

**Extra Curricula Activities:** ______________________________

______________________________

**Health:** ______________________________

______________________________

## Clinical Posting for the MSc Nursing Program

| Month | First Year | Second Year | Remarks |
|---|---|---|---|
| August | | | |
| September | | | |
| October | | | |
| November | | | |
| December | | | |
| January | | | |
| February | | | |
| March | | | |
| April | | | |
| May | | | |
| June | | | |
| July | | | |

**Signature of the Class Coordinator**
**Date:**

**Principal**